The Hidden Dangers of Unexplained Weight Loss

What Your Body Is Trying to Tell You

Sophia Royce Smartwell

DEDICATION

To individuals who work to improve their health, who pay attention to their bodies' subtle cues, and who are committed to learning the truth about the changes they go through. I hope this book helps you on your path to empowerment, healing, and understanding. I would like to express my gratitude to my family, friends, and everyone else who helped me write this work for your unwavering support and conviction in the significance of my message.

Since awareness enables us to make wise decisions and live healthier lives, this book is devoted to those who are interested in learning new things and promoting health.

DISCLAIMER

The Hidden Dangers of Unexplained Weight Loss: What Your Body Is Trying to Tell You contains content that is intended solely for general informational purposes. It is not meant to be a replacement for expert medical guidance, diagnosis, or care. If you have any queries about a medical condition or weight-related issues, you should always consult your doctor or another trained healthcare professional. Nothing in this book should induce you to ignore or put off obtaining expert medical advice.

The publisher and author disclaim all liability for any actions based on the information in this book and make no guarantees or assurances regarding the content's completeness or accuracy. Before adopting any dietary, exercise, or lifestyle changes based on the information presented here, the reader should speak with their healthcare physician.

The information in this book may not be up to date with the latest scientific findings or medical recommendations, as it represents the author's opinions at the time of publishing.

CONTENTS

ACKNOWLEDGMENTS

Without the encouragement and support of many people who believed in this project from the beginning, I could not have finished writing **The Hidden Dangers of Unexplained Weight Loss.** It has been a very gratifying and difficult road.

I want to start by sincerely thanking my family and friends, whose unfailing love, tolerance, and understanding have been a continual source of inspiration for me during this process. Even in times of self-doubt, their confidence in my work has given me the willpower to persevere.

I am also immensely appreciative of the specialists, researchers, and medical professionals who shared their knowledge and perspectives on the complicated subject of inexplicable weight loss. The inspiration for this book came from your efforts and commitment to health and wellbeing. I would especially like to thank the healthcare professionals who so kindly contributed their knowledge and experiences, which enabled me to incorporate their insightful viewpoints into this work.

I want to express my gratitude to my editor and reviewers for their painstaking attention to detail, perceptive criticism, and dedication to making this book the best it can be. Your knowledge and diligence have been really beneficial.

In conclusion, I hope that this book will empower you to take charge of your health, improve your understanding of your body, and inspire you to get the answers you deserve. This book is dedicated to you; may it provide you with the understanding and insight you require on your path to wellbeing.

Thank you.

CHAPTER 1

COMPREHENDING INEXPLICABLE WEIGHT LOSS

Unexpected weight loss may go unreported until it becomes noticeable or interferes with day-to-day functioning, but it can also be an early indicator of underlying health problems. Accurately determining one's health state requires knowledge of this phenomena, including its definition, how to distinguish it from typical fluctuations, and how to spot early warning indicators.

1.1 Overview and Definition

A decrease in body weight that happens without any deliberate or purposeful alteration to one's diet, level of physical activity, or way of life is known as unexplained weight loss. At first, this type of weight loss may not be noticeable, but if it continues or increases over time, it becomes more serious. In contrast to weight loss brought on by diet or exercise, unexplained weight loss may be a sign of a number of illnesses, from gastrointestinal and metabolic disorders to specific types of cancer or mental health issues.

Examining how and why the body loses weight unexpectedly is necessary to comprehend the possible seriousness of unexplained weight loss:

- **Metabolic Factors:** Weight loss without dietary changes might result from infections, hyperthyroidism, or autoimmune illnesses that speed up the body's metabolism.

- The body is unable to retain sufficient calories due to problems with nutrient absorption, such as in Crohn's disease or celiac disease, which results in undesired weight loss.

- **Energy Imbalance:** Stress or hormonal fluctuations may cause the body to spend more energy than it absorbs, which can result in weight loss without conscious effort.

When someone loses more than 5% of their body weight over the course of six to twelve months without a discernible cause, it is typically considered unexplained weight loss in clinical practice. This cutoff point emphasizes the need to keep an eye on even little, inadvertent weight fluctuations since they may be early indicators of more serious health problems.

1.2 Typical Weight Variations versus Weight Loss Concerns

It's critical to distinguish between weight reduction that can indicate health issues and typical, daily weight swings. Weight fluctuates naturally as a result of dietary consumption, physical activity, hormonal fluctuations, and hydration. Usually mild and transient, these variations don't point to a serious health issue.

On the other hand, significant, ongoing weight loss is typically reason for alarm and may be a sign of more serious problems, particularly when linked to the following factors:

- **Duration:** While unexplained weight loss lasts for weeks or months, daily weight fluctuations may go away in 24 to 48 hours.

- **Extent:** While weight reduction is defined as a steady decrease of more than 5% of body weight between six to twelve months, minor changes often fall between 1 and 2 pounds.

- **Associated Symptoms:** Other symptoms related to weight loss, such fever, gastrointestinal distress, weariness, or decreased appetite, may also indicate a particular underlying cause.

Daily variations are frequently linked to natural phenomena such as:

- **Hydration Levels:** Changes in water intake or retention brought on by menstrual cycles, high-sodium foods, or specific drugs.

- **Hormonal Influences:** Hormones, especially insulin

and cortisol, can affect hunger and water retention, leading to slight weight fluctuations.

- **Dietary Changes:** Changes in the amount of salt or carbohydrates consumed, which affect the storage of glycogen and the retention of water.

Knowing these distinctions makes it easier for patients and medical professionals to discern between normal alterations and alarming trends that call for further testing.

1.3 Recognizing Early Indications

Early detection of inexplicable weight loss can help with prompt action and underlying disease diagnosis. These indicators are especially crucial since, if ignored, early, undetected weight loss might result in more serious health problems.

Among the crucial indicators and symptoms of weight loss that cannot be explained are:

- **Short-Term Rapid Weight Loss:** Losing more than 5% of body weight in less than six months, especially if no dietary, lifestyle, or exercise changes are made.

- **Decreased Muscle Mass or Weakness:** Muscle wasting, which is frequently visible in the arms, legs, and face, is a precursor to undesired weight loss brought on by metabolic imbalances or malnutrition.

- The body may not be getting enough nutrition or may be coping with an underlying infection, endocrine condition, or psychological stressor if there is persistent fatigue that comes with weight loss.

- **Change in Appetite or Eating Patterns:** A noticeable decrease in appetite or an early feeling of fullness may be a sign of hormonal changes or gastrointestinal disorders, and it may result in inadvertent weight loss.

- **Digestive Symptoms**: When weight loss is accompanied by bloating, diarrhea, nausea, or stomach discomfort, these symptoms may indicate malabsorption syndromes or digestive diseases.

- **Visible Changes in Physical Appearance:** A noticeable decrease in garment size without conscious effort, along with thinning of the face, neck, or collarbone, can be early signs of inexplicable weight loss.

Early identification and examination of these symptoms enables timely medical assessment, which may help with underlying illness diagnosis and treatment. Healthcare professionals can identify the cause and best course of action for unexplained weight loss by taking a complete approach that includes a physical examination, evaluation of medical history, and potentially laboratory testing.

CHAPTER 2

TYPICAL MEDICAL CONDITIONS ASSOCIATED WITH INEXPLICABLE WEIGHT LOSS

Unexpected weight loss is frequently an indication of underlying medical disorders that interfere with regular body processes and cause nutrient malabsorption or an unexpected calorie deficit. Finding the possible reasons behind inexplicable weight loss can help with early diagnosis and enhance the effectiveness of treatment. This chapter looks at important conditions that are frequently connected to unexpected weight loss and explains how they affect the body.

2.1 The Primary Cause of Cancer

Unaccounted-for weight loss is primarily caused by cancer, especially in its early stages when symptoms are frequently mild. The body's reaction to cancer cells, which can drastically change metabolism and cause a systemic energy imbalance, is usually the cause of this weight loss. Lung, pancreatic, and colon cancers are notable tumors associated with early and inexplicable weight loss.

Weight loss associated with cancer can occur through a number of mechanisms:

1. **Metabolic Changes:** In order to support their quick growth, cancer cells frequently take over the body's energy-production pathways and use nutrients more quickly. Even with a consistent calorie intake, this condition, called cancer cachexia, causes significant weight loss and muscular atrophy.

2. **Inflammation and Cytokine Release:** A lot of malignancies cause the immune system proteins known as inflammatory cytokines to be released, which raises metabolic demand and further exhausts the body's resources. Weight loss and exhaustion are caused by this immunological response, and cytokines may change appetite by making a person feel fuller sooner or less inclined to eat.

3. **Tumor Impact on Organs:** Weight loss may result from direct obstructions to hormone regulation, digestion, or nutrient absorption caused by tumors in

certain organs, such as the pancreas or digestive system.

The Value of Early Diagnosis

The early identification of some malignancies can be greatly aided by unexplained weight loss. Since early diagnosis is frequently associated with better treatment outcomes, patients who have severe weight loss without a clear explanation should have a thorough evaluation. Early cancer detection can increase survival chances, enable less invasive therapies, and possibly slow the disease's spread. Healthcare professionals should therefore closely monitor patients who experience unexplained weight loss and rule out cancer as a potential underlying cause, particularly if it is accompanied by other symptoms like exhaustion, changes in bowel habits, or unexplained pain.

2.2 Intestinal Conditions

Another frequent reason for inexplicable weight loss is gastrointestinal (GI) issues. These illnesses frequently impair the body's capacity to absorb and use nutrients, which over time leads to malnutrition and weight loss.

Celiac disease, persistent diarrhea, and inflammatory bowel diseases (IBD) such as Crohn's disease and ulcerative colitis are important GI conditions linked to inexplicable weight loss.

These gastrointestinal disorders affect how nutrients are absorbed in a number of ways:

1. **Celiac Disease:** This autoimmune condition, which is brought on by eating gluten, damages the small intestine and makes it more difficult for it to absorb nutrients. Even if a person is eating adequate calories, this results in malnutrition.

2. Chronic diarrhea, which is frequently associated with infections or irritable bowel syndrome (IBS), can lead to dehydration and nutrient loss by preventing the intestines from holding onto adequate fluids and nutrients. Additionally, chronic diarrhea shortens the time it takes for food to be absorbed by speeding up its passage through the GI tract.

3. **Inflammatory Bowel Disease (IBD):** Chronic inflammation in the GI tract is caused by diseases such as Crohn's disease and ulcerative colitis. In addition to impairing nutrient absorption and

harming the gut lining, inflammation can cause the body to raise its metabolic rate, which exacerbates weight loss.

Impact on Life Quality and Nutritional Status

Due to malabsorption, people with GI issues frequently experience both weight loss and deficits in vital vitamins and minerals. Complications include anemia, a decline in bone density, and immune system dysfunction may result from this. A multidisciplinary strategy is necessary to treat these diseases, which may involve dietary changes, anti-inflammatory drugs, and occasionally supplements to address deficiencies. Improving the patient's quality of life and preventing severe malnutrition need prompt action.

2.3 Endocrine and Thyroid Conditions

The metabolism can be significantly impacted by thyroid and other endocrine abnormalities, which frequently result in inadvertent weight loss. Through the production of hormones, particularly thyroxine (T4) and triiodothyronine (T3), the thyroid gland plays a vital role in controlling metabolism. Weight, energy levels, and general health can all be impacted by changes in the body's metabolic rate caused by an imbalance in these hormones.

The condition known as hyperthyroidism

The condition known as hyperthyroidism causes the thyroid gland to generate an excessive amount of thyroid hormones, which speeds up the body's metabolism. This elevated metabolic rate raises energy expenditure and frequently causes inadvertent weight loss. Typical signs of hyperthyroidism include:

1. **Increased Appetite with Weight Loss:** Because of their body's faster metabolism, many people with hyperthyroidism may realize that they are eating more but still losing weight.

2. **Heat Intolerance and Sweating:** Excessive sweating and sensitivity to warm temperatures are caused by the body's increased metabolic rate.

3. **Muscle Weakness and weariness:** Even with adequate calorie intake, hyperthyroidism can cause muscle atrophy, which can contribute to weariness and weakness.

Additional Hormonal Disturbances

Unexpected weight loss can also be a symptom of other endocrine conditions such uncontrolled diabetes and adrenal insufficiency (Addison's disease). Cortisol and aldosterone, which are vital for preserving energy levels and metabolic balance, are not produced in sufficient amounts by the adrenal glands in Addison's illness. Fatigue, muscular atrophy, and unintentional weight loss are caused by low cortisol. The body's inability to effectively use glucose, its main energy source, in uncontrolled diabetes causes the body to break down more muscle and fat as it looks for other fuel sources.

Aspects of Diagnosis and Treatment

Blood tests are used to measure hormone levels and contextualize symptoms in order to diagnose thyroid and endocrine problems. Radioactive iodine therapy, hormone-level-regulating drugs, and, in extreme situations, surgery are all possible treatments for hyperthyroidism. Targeted hormone replacement treatment or medication can assist restore metabolic equilibrium and stop more weight loss for other hormonal abnormalities.

CHAPTER 3

MENTAL HEALTH'S CONTRIBUTION TO INEXPLICABLE

WEIGHT LOSS

A person's weight is significantly influenced by their mental wellbeing. Mental health issues are frequently the primary or contributing reason in cases of unexplained weight loss. A number of physiological and psychological processes linked to mental health disorders can influence metabolism, eating habits, and hunger, all of which can have an effect on weight. This chapter explores the situations and causes that may impact weight changes in people dealing with psychological issues, delving into the complex relationship between mental health and unexplained weight loss.

3.1 Disorders of Anxiety and Depression

Two of the most prevalent mental health issues in the world, anxiety and depression, can have a major impact on eating habits and appetite, frequently resulting in unwanted weight loss. The way the body processes food and the urge to eat can be affected by any of these conditions, which can interfere with normal physical functions and emotional reactions.

Depression

A persistently down mood, hopelessness, and a lack of drive or energy are common symptoms of depression. Eating habits and other aspects of everyday life may be significantly impacted by these symptoms. Depression frequently causes people to lose their appetite or become disinterested in eating completely, which over time may result in inadvertent weight loss. Among the contributing elements are:

- **Loss of Pleasure in Eating:** Also referred to as anhedonia, this condition is characterized by a diminished capacity to experience pleasure in eating and other activities. Food may no longer taste good to some people, which causes them to consume less calories.

- **Fatigue and Low Energy**: Depression frequently results in extreme exhaustion, which, in extreme situations, makes cooking or eating seem impossible. People may thus skip meals or eat less food in general.

- **Physiological Changes:** Depression can suppress hunger signals and reduce calorie intake because it affects the hypothalamus, a part of the brain that controls appetite and metabolism.

Apprehension

Anxiety disorders, such as panic disorder, social anxiety disorder, and generalized anxiety disorder, can affect eating habits and cause weight loss. Increased anxiety triggers the "fight-or-flight" reaction in the body, which raises cortisol and adrenaline levels, which can affect metabolism and appetite. Anxiety-related weight loss is largely caused by:

- Eating can become difficult or undesirable due to gastrointestinal problems like nausea, stomachaches, or indigestion, which are frequently brought on by anxiety.

- **Increased Caloric Expenditure:** Even in the absence of changes in physical activity, the body's reaction to worry involves an increase in heart rate and metabolic rate, which results in a higher energy expenditure.

- **Disrupted Eating Patterns:** People who suffer from anxiety may eat sporadically or avoid meals because they are anxious or worried, which results in irregular calorie intake.

Chronic Stress

Overeating can occasionally result from stress, but chronic stress can also make some people less hungry. Prolonged stress causes cortisol levels to rise, which can interfere with hunger signals and digestion, leading to weight loss. Chronic stress also has a detrimental effect on sleep, which can exacerbate weight loss by impairing metabolism and making people feel more exhausted.

Determining and Treating Weight Loss in Anxiety and Depression

When treating individuals who are losing weight for no apparent reason, medical professionals should think about doing an anxiety and depression assessment. Cognitive-behavioral therapy (CBT) is one intervention that may be used to enhance appetite and emotional control. In certain situations, medication may also be used.

By suggesting nutrient-dense, simple-to-make foods that satisfy calorie requirements and compensate for nutrient shortages, dieticians and nutritionists can also assist patients.

3.2 Weight Loss and Eating Disorders

Unhealthy eating patterns and behaviors are closely linked to eating disorders, a serious category of mental health issues that frequently cause substantial weight loss. In some situations, weight loss is an indirect result of disordered eating patterns, while in others, it may be deliberate in diseases such as anorexia. Healthcare professionals must have a thorough understanding of these illnesses since early intervention can enhance recovery and avoid consequences.

Neurosa anorexia

Severe food restriction, a distorted body image, and an overwhelming fear of gaining weight are the hallmarks of anorexia nervosa. To prevent weight gain, people with anorexia may exercise excessively or follow strict food restrictions. Among the effects of anorexia are:

- **Severe Malnutrition:** When calorie intake is restricted, malnutrition results in nutritional shortages, which impair organ function and weaken the immune system.

- **Physical Health Risks:** Anorexia can lead to heart arrhythmias, muscle atrophy, brittle bones, and in extreme situations, multi-organ failure.

- **Psychological Factors:** Anorexia is frequently linked to perfectionism and high levels of self-criticism, which reinforce restrictive eating habits.

Nervosa bulimia

Episodes of binge eating followed by compensatory behaviors, such vomiting, excessive exercise, or using laxatives to "purge" the calories consumed, are characteristics of bulimia nervosa. Bulimia sufferers may not necessarily lose a lot of weight, but those who purge often run the danger of dehydration, electrolyte imbalances, and nutritional deficiencies, all of which can cause inexplicable weight loss.

Disordered Eating Patterns, Including Binge Eating

Disorder

Individuals with binge-eating disorder do not purge; instead, they ingest massive quantities of food in a little period of time. Weight fluctuations, however, might result from mental strain and irregular eating habits that interfere with regular metabolic functions. Unintended weight loss may also be caused by other disordered eating practices, such as orthorexia (an obsession with "healthy") and restrictive eating.

Impact on General Health and the Requirement for All-Inclusive Care

Because eating disorders are complicated, a multimodal approach to treatment is necessary, involving medical monitoring, dietary counseling, and psychotherapy. Because these diseases can have long-lasting impacts on one's bodily and mental health, early intervention is crucial. Stabilizing weight, addressing nutritional deficiencies, and addressing the psychological aspects that underlie disordered eating patterns are the main objectives of treatment.

3.3 Changes in Appetite and Medication

Prescription drugs for mental health issues, especially mood stabilizers, antidepressants, and antipsychotics, can have adverse effects that affect taste, appetite, and metabolism, which can result in unexpected weight fluctuations. Some drugs may suppress appetite or change dietary preferences, which can lead to weight loss, while others are more likely to induce weight gain.

Antidepressants

People who take some antidepressants, particularly selective serotonin reuptake inhibitors (SSRIs), may experience nausea or decreased appetite, which makes it harder for them to consume enough calories. Antidepressant side effects that frequently result in weight loss include:

- **Nausea and Digestive Discomfort:** Nausea is a typical initial adverse effect that can decrease appetite, but it usually gets better as the body becomes used to the drug.

- **Altered Taste and Smell:** Some people claim that food tastes different or less appetizing, which can make them less inclined to eat.

Medications for Stimulants

Often taken for disorders such as ADHD, stimulant medicines have the potential to drastically decrease appetite. Dopamine and norepinephrine levels are raised by stimulants, which might reduce appetite and cause weight reduction. To compensate for decreased appetite, patients taking these drugs might require advice on how to plan nutrient-dense meals.

Medications for Antipsychotics

Depending on the patient and the particular antipsychotic, some antipsychotics might cause weight gain or loss. While certain antipsychotics may cause metabolic changes that lead to weight gain, others may have a calming effect that decreases appetite and physical activity. Working with a healthcare professional to monitor and modify antipsychotic medication can help prevent unexpected weight fluctuations.

Methods for Handling Weight Shifts Caused by Drugs

When taking medicine that alters appetite, patients should

speak with their doctor about other options, dosage modifications, or other weight-management strategies. Increased consumption of small, nutrient-dense meals is one dietary strategy that can help offset unexpected weight loss. Healthcare professionals can assist patients in identifying alternatives that strike a balance between weight stability and mental health advantages, and some drugs have less appetite-suppressing side effects.

Effectively identifying and managing unexplained weight loss requires an understanding of the relationship between weight and mental health. Healthcare professionals can develop all-encompassing treatment programs that promote mental and physical health and aid in long-term rehabilitation and well-being by recognizing and addressing mental health problems.

CHAPTER 4

Unexpected Weight Loss in Older Adults

In older adults, unexplained weight loss is a serious worry since it frequently points to underlying medical conditions that need immediate care. Since weight loss in older people is often linked to higher rates of morbidity and mortality, it is critical to comprehend, identify, and promptly address this issue. This chapter explores age-related risk factors, the prevalence of unexplained weight loss in older persons, and the significance of screening and intervention in preventing serious health outcomes.

4.1 Prevalence in Environments of Community Living

Older persons frequently experience unexplained weight loss, especially those who live in nursing homes or assisted living facilities. According to research, older persons who lose weight had higher hospitalization rates, higher levels of reliance, and a lower quality of life. Physical, social, and environmental variables specific to this demographic often contribute to the incidence of unexplained weight loss in these contexts.

Data on Weight Loss in the Elderly

According to studies, between 15% and 20% of senior citizens lose a considerable amount of weight each year without intending to. In institutional settings, where up to 50% of nursing home residents lose weight over time, the prevalence is significantly higher. The complicated medical requirements of senior citizens and the particular difficulties of managing several chronic illnesses in such environments are contributing factors to this high frequency.

Contributing Elements in Social Environments

Unexpected weight loss in older individuals can be caused by a number of community living-specific factors:

- **Dietary Limitations:** Residents' appetites and food intake may be diminished by meals at these facilities that are bland, unappealing, or inadequately nutrient-dense.
- **Social Isolation:** In communal settings, older

persons may feel lonely or unsociable, which might influence their appetite and lead to a decrease in calorie intake.

- **Medical Complexity:** Elderly residents in nursing homes frequently have a number of comorbid conditions and drugs that interact in ways that affect their ability to eat, digest, and absorb nutrients.

The necessity for specific dietary and social interventions to improve nutritional health is highlighted by the high prevalence of weight loss among older persons in these settings. Proactively addressing these variables can enhance health outcomes and stop the decrease brought on by inadvertent weight loss.

4.2 Risk Factors Associated with Age

Due to physiological changes brought on by aging, older persons are more susceptible to accidental weight loss. Predisposing older persons to weight loss and nutritional problems is largely due to age-related variables, such as decreased appetite, hormonal changes, muscle loss, and chronic illnesses. Healthcare professionals, caregivers, and family members must be aware of these risk factors in order to spot weight loss symptoms early and take the proper action.

Muscle Mass Loss

Sarcopenia, or the progressive loss of muscle mass that comes with aging, is a major contributing factor to weight loss in older persons. In addition to lowering body weight, sarcopenia affects physical function, making it more difficult for elderly people to remain mobile and independent. Because muscle tissue is metabolically active and burns calories even while at rest, muscle loss has an impact on metabolism. The body needs less energy when there is less muscle, which lowers hunger and calorie intake.

Decreased Appetite and Taste and Smell Changes

As people age, their appetite naturally decreases; this is referred to as "anorexia of aging." Age-related changes in taste and scent can also lead to a decrease in appetite. Food intake may decline in older persons because they find it less enticing and pleasurable. Among the main causes of elderly persons' decreased appetite are:

- **Hormonal Changes:** As people age, their levels of hunger-regulating hormones, such as ghrelin and leptin, may become unbalanced, which lessens sensations of hunger.

- **Medications:** A lot of drugs that are frequently provided to elderly patients, like blood pressure drugs, antidepressants, and painkillers, might change taste or decrease appetite.

Comorbidities and Chronic Illnesses

Chronic illnesses that affect dietary intake and nutrient absorption, such as diabetes, dementia, cardiovascular disease, and respiratory problems, are prevalent in older persons. Eating can be difficult when chronic illnesses cause symptoms like discomfort, nausea, or trouble swallowing. Additionally, a lot of older folks deal with several diseases, which makes eating more difficult and can make losing weight more difficult. A comprehensive approach to food planning is necessary when there are several chronic illnesses present because each one may have different dietary requirements and constraints.

Health Issues with the Mind

Eating habits are greatly impacted by mental health issues, which are prevalent in older persons, including depression and cognitive impairment. Depression in older adults frequently takes a different form than in younger people; it can show itself as weariness, indifference, or a loss of appetite. Unintentional weight loss may result from cognitive decline, such as Alzheimer's disease and other types of dementia, which can affect a person's capacity to detect hunger cues or remember to eat.

4.3 Intervention and Screening

Effective management of this issue requires routine screening and prompt action due to the high prevalence of unexplained weight loss in older persons and the health hazards involved. Early identification of weight loss in senior citizens can enhance quality of life and stop additional health decline.

The Value of Frequent Weight Checks

A vital component of care for senior citizens, particularly those living in community settings, is routine weight monitoring. If unexplained weight loss is noticed, weight checks can lead to additional research and serve as an early warning sign of possible health problems. The following elements should be taken into account by healthcare professionals when tracking weight:

- **Frequency:** For older people, particularly those who are at risk of malnutrition or have chronic conditions, weight should ideally be monitored weekly or at least monthly.

- **Consistency:** To guarantee accuracy and identify minute variations, measurements should be made with the same scale, at the same time of day, and in comparable circumstances.

Checking for Root Reasons

A thorough evaluation is required to determine possible causes if unexplained weight loss is found. The following should be screened:

- **Medical Evaluation:** Checking for gastrointestinal problems, infections, or chronic illnesses that could be causing weight loss.

- **Mental Health Assessment:** Examining for symptoms of anxiety, depression, or cognitive decline that may affect eating habits and appetite.

- **Medication Review:** Examining the patient's prescriptions for adverse effects that could impair digestion or decrease appetite.

Nutritional and Dietary Interventions

Dietary interventions can be used to promote healthy weight maintenance when the root causes of weight loss have been determined. Providing nutrient-dense foods that are simple to prepare and eat should be the main goal of nutrition initiatives for senior citizens. Important strategies consist of:

- **Caloric and Protein Fortification:** Including foods high in calories and protein in meals, such as lean meats, eggs, and full-fat dairy, can assist older persons maintain their energy levels and muscle mass.

- **Small, Frequent Meals:** Providing smaller, more frequent meals can help people regulate their eating habits and increase their overall calorie intake, particularly for individuals who have a decreased appetite.

- **Taste and Texture Modification:** Food accessibility and attractiveness can be enhanced for people with taste or chewing issues by using flavor-enhancing additives or by modifying textures (such purees or softer foods).

Enhancing the Environment and Society

Creating a welcoming and social mealtime atmosphere might positively affect appetite and food intake in communal living environments. Eating with people can improve the mealtime experience and promote food consumption, according to studies. Among the environmental changes made to enhance the dining experience are:

- **Social Meal Settings:** Promoting communal meals and offering company to promote a feeling of community.

- **Appealing Presentation:** To improve satisfaction and pique desire, meals should be presented with attention to visual appeal and variation in flavors and colors.

Pharmacological and Medical Interventions

In certain situations, older adults may require pharmaceutical or medical measures to help them maintain their weight. Each person's health profile should be taken into account when choosing from these possibilities. Among the possible interventions are:

- **Appetite Stimulants:** In situations when extreme weight loss is affecting health, doctors may prescribe certain drugs, such as megestrol acetate, to increase appetite.

- **Nutritional Supplements:** For people who have trouble eating regular meals, protein shakes, vitamin supplements, or specifically made liquids can assist meet nutritional needs.

In order to find and treat the underlying reasons of older individuals' unexplained weight loss, a thorough, customized approach is necessary. The health and well-being of older persons can be supported by healthcare professionals, caregivers, and family members working together to identify age-related risk factors, assess the prevalence of this issue, and implement timely interventions.

CHAPTER 5

METABOLIC AND GASTROINTESTINAL DISORDERS AFFECTING WEIGHT

One of the main reasons for inexplicable weight loss is metabolic and gastrointestinal (GI) disorders. These illnesses may impair the body's capacity to maintain regular metabolic functions, control hunger, and absorb vital nutrients. This chapter explores the ways in which metabolic disorders like diabetes and metabolic syndrome, conditions like celiac disease and inflammatory bowel disease (IBD), chronic diarrhea, and malabsorption problems all contribute to unintended weight loss, which frequently results in major health complications if left untreated.

5.1 Malabsorption and Prolonged Diarrhea

Malabsorption and chronic diarrhea are two associated disorders that can have a major effect on body weight and frequently result in unwanted weight loss. These illnesses make it difficult for the body to absorb the nutrients it needs from food, which can lead to severe weight loss, dehydration, and nutritional deficiencies.

Chronic Diarrhea and Loss of Nutrients

Frequent, loose, or watery stools are known as diarrhea, and they can be caused by a number of underlying illnesses, such as infections, inflammatory diseases, and certain drugs. Chronic diarrhea, which lasts for weeks or months, can cause a substantial loss of nutrients and interfere with the absorption of vital vitamins and minerals.

Fluid and Electrolyte Imbalance: Dehydration, which happens when the body loses too many fluids and electrolytes, is one of the direct consequences of chronic diarrhea. Although it is mostly caused by fluid loss rather than loss of muscle or fat, dehydration can cause a decrease in body weight.

- **nutritional Deficiencies:** Diarrhea speeds up the passage of food through the intestines, which hinders adequate nutritional absorption and digestion. Important nutrients, such as proteins, minerals, and fat-soluble vitamins A, D, E, and K, may not be absorbed in enough amounts, leading to shortages that can exacerbate weight loss.

Malabsorption Conditions

The term "malabsorption" describes the gastrointestinal tract's compromised capacity to absorb nutrients from meals, which can result in weight loss, persistent diarrhea, and other symptoms including gas and bloating. The following effects can result from conditions that interfere with the normal absorption process, such as celiac disease, chronic pancreatitis, and specific infections:

- **Malabsorption of Fat:** Steatorrhea, or fatty feces, are caused when the body is unable to adequately absorb fat. These stools can be large, smell bad, and be challenging to pass. Since lipids are a major source of calories and energy, this condition frequently results in unintended weight loss.

- **Malabsorption of Proteins and Carbohydrates:** Proteins and carbs are essential energy sources, just like lipids. Fatigue, muscular atrophy, and severe weight loss can be caused by inadequate absorption of certain macronutrients.

Treating the underlying causes—whether they be infections, long-term illnesses, or digestive disorders—is essential to managing chronic diarrhea and malabsorption. To lessen symptoms and enhance nutrient absorption, dietary changes, enzyme replacement therapy, or prescription drugs may be necessary in certain situations.

5.2 Inflammatory Bowel Disease and Celiac Disease

Two chronic gastrointestinal disorders that cause severe inflammation, malabsorption, and unexpected weight loss include celiac disease and inflammatory bowel disease (IBD). A number of gastrointestinal symptoms, such as persistent diarrhea, abdominal pain, and bloating, are brought on by these disorders, which interfere with proper digestion and can result in inadequate nutrition and weight loss.

Celiac Disease

Gluten, a protein included in wheat, barley, and rye, causes an immunological reaction that harms the lining of the small intestine in people with celiac disease, an autoimmune condition. Over time, this damage might result in severe weight loss because it hinders the absorption of vital nutrients. Celiac disease can cause systemic symptoms like exhaustion and skin rashes in addition to gastrointestinal problems.

The small intestine's villi, which are microscopic projections that resemble hairs, are attacked by the immune system in persons with celiac disease, which hinders their ability to absorb nutrients. As a result, important minerals like iron, calcium, and fat-soluble vitamins A, D, E, and K are not properly absorbed, which can lead to weight loss and other issues including osteoporosis and anemia.

The immune system's inflammatory reaction to gluten causes bloating, diarrhea, and cramping in the abdomen, among other symptoms. The disease-related weight loss is made worse by the persistent inflammation, which also interferes with digestion and absorption.

Following a rigorous gluten-free diet is essential for managing celiac disease because it promotes intestinal healing and better nutritional absorption. People with celiac disease can frequently regain lost weight and enhance their general health if diagnosed early and treated appropriately.

IBD, or Inflammatory Bowel Disease

IBD includes diseases that cause persistent inflammation of the gastrointestinal system, such as Crohn's disease and ulcerative colitis. Both illnesses can cause severe weight loss by affecting distinct regions of the intestines and causing symptoms like lethargy, bloody stools, diarrhea, and abdominal pain.

Any region of the gastrointestinal tract may be impacted by Crohn's disease, which is characterized by erratic flare-ups. Crohn's disease-induced inflammation reduces the absorption of nutrients, particularly in the small intestine. People may lose weight as a result of hunger and elevated energy expenditure brought on by persistent inflammation.

- **Colitis Ulcerative:** Although the colon is the primary site of ulcerative colitis, the intestinal lining becomes inflamed and ulcerated as well, resulting in symptoms that resemble those of Crohn's disease. Common symptoms include cramping in the abdomen, blood in the stool, and diarrhea, which can lead to dehydration and weight loss.

Malnutrition can arise from poor nutrient absorption brought on by inflammation, elevated metabolic needs, and decreased appetite in both Crohn's disease and ulcerative colitis. Anti-inflammatory drugs, immune system suppressors, and occasionally surgery to remove afflicted intestinal segments are all possible treatments for IBD.

5.3 Metabolic Syndrome and Diabetes

Metabolic disorders including diabetes and metabolic syndrome can have complicated effects on appetite, body weight, and nutrition absorption. Unintentional weight loss is a common consequence of both illnesses, frequently brought on by insulin resistance, poor blood sugar regulation, and disturbed metabolic processes.

Diabetes and Loss of Weight

Despite eating more food, uncontrolled diabetes, especially type 1 and advanced type 2, can cause severe weight loss. There are multiple explanations for this weight loss:

- **Insulin Deficiency or Resistance:** Insulin, a

hormone that aids cells in absorbing glucose for energy, is not produced by the body in people with type 1 diabetes. Insulin resistance develops in people with type 2 diabetes. In both situations, the body breaks down fat and muscle for energy instead of using glucose as it should when insulin activity is inadequate. This leads to inadvertent weight loss.

- **Dehydration and Increased urine:** Diabetes's elevated blood sugar levels cause the body to lose fluids through increased urine. Although dehydration is the main cause, weight loss can also result from fluid loss.

- **nutritional Loss:** The body may expel more glucose through the urine if it is not taken into the cells, which can result in nutritional imbalances and more weight loss.

Effectively controlling blood sugar levels, lowering excessive urination, and avoiding the severe weight loss frequently linked to diabetes can all be achieved with appropriate insulin administration, nutrition, and exercise.

Weight Loss and Metabolic Syndrome

The metabolic syndrome is a group of diseases that raise the risk of heart disease, stroke, and type 2 diabetes. These conditions include high blood pressure, raised blood sugar, extra abdominal fat, and abnormal cholesterol levels. Although weight increase is usually linked to metabolic syndrome, it can also result in weight reduction in certain situations, especially if the illness is poorly treated.

The metabolic syndrome is characterized by insulin resistance, which might hinder the body's capacity to retain and utilize glucose. Weight loss may result from the body burning muscle and fat for energy.

- **Fatty Liver Disease:** Weight loss may also be a result of non-alcoholic fatty liver disease (NAFLD), which is frequently observed in people with metabolic syndrome. Damage to the liver impairs the body's capacity to absorb nutrients, which can result in malabsorption and weight loss.

Reversing or lessening the symptoms of metabolic syndrome and avoiding unexpected weight loss need early intervention and lifestyle changes like eating better, exercising more, and controlling blood sugar levels.

By interfering with proper digestion, nutritional absorption, and metabolic control, gastrointestinal and metabolic disorders can have a substantial effect on weight. Effective weight loss management and the avoidance of long-term health issues depend on an understanding of the mechanisms behind these disorders and how they affect body weight. Healthcare providers can help people with these problems regain their health and stop more weight loss by treating the underlying reasons and offering appropriate therapies.

CHAPTER 6

FINANCIAL AND SOCIAL ASPECTS OF INEXPLICABLE WEIGHT LOSS

In addition to physical and medical issues, social and financial variables are also implicated in unexplained weight loss. A person's capacity to maintain a healthy weight can be greatly impacted by physical limitations, financial stress, social isolation, and restricted access to food. This chapter examines the ways in which these financial and societal factors lead to unexpected weight loss, especially in vulnerable groups like the elderly, those with impairments, and those with low incomes.

6.1 Limited Resources and Food Insecurity

One important socioeconomic element causing unexplained weight loss is food insecurity, which is characterized as the inability to consistently obtain enough nutrient-dense food for an active and healthy life.

Malnutrition, undernutrition, and weight loss can result from a person's inability to buy enough food due to financial strain, unemployment, and other economic difficulties.

The Effects of Financial Stress

Food may become less important to many people who are struggling financially when they prioritize necessities like shelter, healthcare, and utilities. In these situations, people and families may find it challenging to buy adequate food, especially nutrient-dense and healthful ones, due to a lack of funds or resources.

Limited Access to Healthy Food: Even when food is reasonably priced, it could be processed and not contain the nutrients needed to maintain a healthy weight. For instance, residents of food deserts regions with limited access to wholesome food and fresh produce may be compelled to rely on inexpensive, high-calorie foods that are insufficiently nutritious.

- **Suboptimal Food Choices:** People may choose inexpensive, satisfying foods that are frequently low in nutrients and heavy in empty calories due to financial pressure to stretch their limited means. If the body cannot get enough energy from these meals, this kind of diet might eventually result in vitamin deficiencies, digestive problems, and inadvertent weight loss.

Populations at Risk

Food insecurity is particularly dangerous for some groups. These include elderly people on fixed incomes, low-income families, and people with long-term medical issues that make financial burden worse. For instance:

- **Elderly People:** A large number of senior persons have fixed incomes and little access to financial resources. They might also experience mental and physical health issues that make food preparation and purchasing more challenging.

- Economically disadvantaged families frequently find it difficult to feed their children a healthy diet, which can cause growth delays and unintended weight loss in youngsters.

Systemic measures are needed to combat food insecurity, including expanding access to food assistance programs, supporting food banks, and enhancing the availability and affordability of wholesome meals in underprivileged areas.

6.2 The Impact of Isolation on Appetite

Eating habits, appetite, and weight can all be significantly impacted by social isolation, especially in older adults. Living alone and not having frequent social interactions can make many older persons less inclined to cook or eat regular, well-balanced meals. This may eventually lead to malnourishment and inexplicable weight loss.

Isolation's Psychological Impact

Depression, loneliness, and a loss of interest in everyday tasks, such as eating, can result from social isolation. Reduced appetite and disinterest in food are frequently associated with depression and bad mood, which can lead to weight loss. Furthermore, meals may seem less meaningful when there is seldom social connection, such as eating with family or friends, which lowers the desire to eat.

Depression and Loss of Appetite: Depression affects a lot of people who are lonely, and it can make it difficult for them to cook or eat. In addition, depression can cause gastrointestinal problems such as constipation, bloating, and nausea, all of which lead to a reduction in food consumption.

- **Lack of Motivation to Eat:** Older folks may start skipping meals or neglect to prepare wholesome meals if they don't have support from their families or friends. The person may not receive the social cues that might ordinarily encourage them to eat at regular intervals as a result of the absence of engagement.

Practical and Physical Obstacles to Eating

Physical restrictions that make eating more challenging are also frequently associated with social isolation. For instance, older people living alone could struggle to prepare meals or have mobility issues that keep them from going grocery shopping or participating in community food programs.

Meal Preparation Difficulties: People may find it challenging to prepare meals due to physical limitations such as arthritis, diminished muscle strength, or cognitive decline. They might turn to fast, unhealthy food options or skip meals entirely as a result.

- **Cognitive Decline:** Cognitive impairments like dementia or Alzheimer's disease can sometimes cause people to forget to eat or struggle to understand the significance of nutrition, which makes weight loss even more difficult.

6.3 Physical Obstacles to Obtaining Food

Another important factor in inexplicable weight loss is physical obstacles to food access, particularly for people with disabilities or long-term medical issues. These obstacles may make it more difficult for someone to get, prepare, or eat food, which could result in poor nutrition and weight loss.

Dysphagia, or difficulty swallowing

Many older people and people with neurological conditions like Parkinson's disease or stroke suffer from dysphagia, which is the inability to swallow. People who have dysphagia may have trouble swallowing liquids and solid foods, which can result in aspiration pneumonia, choking, or just a dislike of eating because it hurts.

Inadequate nourishment: Individuals who have dysphagia may only be able to eat soft or pureed foods that don't provide enough nourishment, or they may avoid foods that are hard to swallow. As the person's caloric intake declines over time, this may lead to noticeable weight loss.

- **Choking and Fear of Eating:** People who are afraid of choking may limit their food intake, which can make mealtimes stressful. This may lessen the frequency of meals and make weight loss even more difficult.

Reduced Mobility and Physical Disabilities

Accessing food is extremely difficult for people with physical limitations or decreased mobility. These obstacles could be related to transportation, meal preparation, or getting to grocery stores. Without the right support, kids can rely on processed, less nutrient-dense foods or miss meals entirely.

- **Limited Access to Food Stores:** If grocery stores or food banks are far away or there aren't many public transportation choices, people with mobility issues may find it difficult to get there.

- **Difficulty in Meal Preparation:** People who have physical limitations, including joint discomfort or paralysis, may find it difficult to cook on their own. Additionally, they might not be physically capable of carrying goods or cooking complicated meals, which could lead to malnourishment and weight loss.

Changes Associated with Age

Physical changes brought on by aging, such as diminished taste perception, decreased appetite, or trouble chewing and digesting food, can make eating habits even more challenging. For instance:

- **Decreased Appetite in the senior**: Aging, hormonal changes, or decreased physical activity can all cause a natural decrease in appetite in many senior people, which can lead to inadvertent weight loss.

- **Dental Issues:** Eating can become painful and challenging due to problems like tooth loss or poorly fitting dentures, which can result in less food being consumed and, in certain situations, severe weight loss.

The development of inexplicable weight loss, especially in vulnerable groups, is significantly influenced by social and socioeconomic circumstances. It can be challenging for people to maintain a healthy weight when normal eating patterns are disrupted by food instability, isolation, and physical impediments to food access. Improving access to wholesome food, offering social support, and addressing the physical obstacles that prevent eating are all important components of a multidimensional strategy to address these problems. Healthcare professionals can help people prevent and manage inexplicable weight loss by identifying and addressing these socioeconomic determinants of health.

CHAPTER 7

A complicated clinical problem, unexplained weight loss is commonly described as the loss of 5% or more of total body weight over a period of 6–12 months without a deliberate change in diet or exercise. Psychosocial issues and severe medical disorders are among the possible explanations. Finding the root reason of inexplicable weight loss is essential to treating the condition effectively and averting other issues. The diagnostic procedure, standard testing and imaging methods, and the value of a multidisciplinary approach to guarantee a thorough and accurate diagnosis are all covered in this chapter.

7.1 The Process of Diagnosis

A comprehensive medical evaluation that includes a history, a physical examination, and potentially more research is the first step in the diagnosis procedure for unexplained weight loss. Given that weight loss is frequently vague and can be caused by a number of illnesses, medical professionals usually take a methodical approach to identifying the underlying reason for this symptom.

Taking History

Getting a thorough medical history from the patient is the first step in the diagnostic procedure. To learn more about the patient's daily routine, lifestyle factors, and weight loss pattern, a healthcare professional will pose targeted inquiries. Important elements of taking a history include:

Duration and Pattern of Weight Loss: It's critical to comprehend the rate of weight loss and if it has been consistent or sporadic. While progressive weight loss may be more suggestive of chronic diseases or metabolic problems, rapid weight loss over a brief period of time frequently indicates an urgent medical crisis.

- **Dietary Habits and Appetite:** Finding disorders that impact food intake, such as anorexia, depression, or gastrointestinal disorders, can be aided by evaluating the patient's appetite and eating habits. A thorough food journal or a conversation about recent dietary adjustments can yield important hints.

- **Psychosocial Factors:** Unintentional weight loss may be associated with mental health conditions such anxiety or depression, stress, and social isolation. Important psychological factors can be identified by inquiring about significant life experiences or changes in lifestyle.

- Inquiring about any history of chronic illnesses, drug use, or recent hospitalizations is crucial because conditions like diabetes, heart disease, or cancer can have a substantial impact on weight.

- **Family History:** Hereditary problems that may be causing weight loss may be indicated by a family history of cancer, gastrointestinal disorders, or autoimmune disorders.

Physical Inspection

A physical examination is conducted after a comprehensive history is taken in order to evaluate the patient's overall health and spot any symptoms that might point to the reason for weight loss. Important components of the test consist of:

- **Vital Signs:** Temperature, heart rate, and blood pressure readings can all offer crucial information. For instance, a low blood pressure result may be a sign of dehydration, malnourishment, or hormonal abnormalities, but a fever may signal an infection or cancer.

- A physical examination determines the degree of muscular atrophy and weight loss (cachexia), which can be observed in diseases including cancer, persistent infections, or malnutrition. Additionally, clinicians may look for symptoms of malnutrition, such as hair loss, brittle nails, and dry skin.

- Tenderness, bloating, or indications of underlying disorders such as pancreatic disease, neurological dysfunction, or inflammatory bowel disease can be found during a focused abdominal and neurological examination if gastrointestinal problems or neurological conditions are suspected.

7.2 Typical Examinations and Imaging Methods

Diagnostic testing and imaging methods are used to narrow down the possible causes of unexplained weight loss when a healthcare provider has obtained enough information through a history and physical examination. These tests aid in the detection of conditions that a physical examination might not be able to reveal right away.

Blood tests

Since blood tests offer important information about an individual's general health and organ function, they are frequently the first line of inquiry for unexplained weight loss. Among the important blood tests that could be requested are:

- Anemia, infections, and some blood malignancies (such leukemia or lymphoma) that can cause weight loss can all be found using a complete blood count (CBC). Low hemoglobin levels can also be a sign of malnutrition or chronic sickness.

- **Thyroid Function Tests:** Hyperthyroidism, a disorder that speeds up metabolism and can lead to weight loss, can be indicated by low thyroid-stimulating hormone (TSH) levels and elevated thyroid hormones (T3 and T4). On the other hand, hypothyroidism, which can occasionally result in mild weight swings, may be indicated by low thyroid hormone levels.

- **Renal Function and Electrolyte Tests:** These tests look for metabolic abnormalities, renal dysfunction, or dehydration symptoms that could cause unexpected weight loss.

- Abnormal liver enzymes can be a sign of bile duct obstruction or liver illness, both of which can cause weight loss.

- **Infection or Inflammation Markers:** Elevated C-reactive protein (CRP) or erythrocyte sedimentation rate (ESR) values could indicate an autoimmune condition, underlying infection, or inflammatory process that is causing weight loss.

- **Cancer Markers:** Although these are usually used in combination with other diagnostic methods, some blood tests can measure cancer-specific markers, such as CEA (carcinoembryonic antigen) for colorectal cancer or CA 19-9 for pancreatic cancer.

Tests for Urine

Another popular diagnostic method is urine testing, which is especially useful for identifying symptoms of renal illness or diabetes. For example:

- **Urinalysis:** This test can detect glucose in the urine, a sign of uncontrolled diabetes, which can cause weight loss.
- A 24-hour urine collection can be used to measure kidney function and look for indications of chronic renal disease or malabsorption.

Imaging Methods

Imaging scans are crucial for identifying functional or structural problems that can be causing weight loss. These instruments offer a non-invasive means of examining the body and identifying anomalies. Typical imaging methods consist of:

- Although chest X-rays are typically not the first option for detecting unexplained weight loss, they can aid in the detection of lung conditions such as cancer, pneumonia, or tuberculosis, all of which can cause weight loss.

- The liver, pancreas, gallbladder, and kidneys can all be affected by disorders that can be detected by an abdominal ultrasound. Finding tumors, inflammation, or blockages that may be causing weight loss is made easier with this.

- **CT Scan:** A computed tomography (CT) scan helps detect cancers, infections, and inflammatory disorders by providing comprehensive images of the chest, abdomen, and other organs.

- **MRI:** MRI provides high-resolution pictures of soft tissues and can be helpful in identifying problems that are causing weight loss in the brain, spine, or abdomen, such as tumors, brain lesions, or nerve damage.

7.3 Using Multidisciplinary Methods to Diagnose

Because there are so many possible reasons for inexplicable weight loss, a multidisciplinary approach is frequently necessary to guarantee a thorough and precise diagnosis. In order to determine the underlying cause of the illness, this strategy entails cooperation amongst multiple medical professionals, each of whom contributes knowledge in a distinct field.

Nutritionists and Dietitians

When it comes to detecting and treating unexplained weight loss, dietitians and nutritionists are frequently crucial, particularly when the problem is linked to malnutrition or bad eating habits. They can uncover any deficiencies or problems with gastrointestinal malabsorption, suggest dietary changes, and assist in determining the patient's nutritional status.

- A dietitian will perform a comprehensive nutritional assessment, taking into account food consumption, portion sizes, and any obstacles to eating. To assess nutritional intake, they might also employ instruments like a 24-hour recall or meal journal.
- In the event that malnutrition is detected, the dietitian will create a customized nutrition plan that includes suggestions for dietary modifications or supplements to help maintain weight.

Both psychiatrists and psychologists

When it comes to assessing weight loss caused by

psychological problems like eating disorders, anxiety, or depression, mental health practitioners are essential. Psychologists and psychiatrists can ascertain whether weight loss is a sign of a psychological disorder rather than a merely medical one by doing a mental health evaluation.

- **Evaluating Mental Health:** Psychological assessments assist in identifying if the patient's weight loss is related to disorders like depression, bulimia, or anorexia, or to emotional distress or disordered eating patterns.

- **Therapeutic Interventions:** Therapy, counseling, or medication may be used to address the underlying problem if a psychological aspect is causing weight loss.

Experts

Referrals to experts may be required to look into particular conditions further, depending on the results of the initial tests and the history taken. The following experts could be involved in diagnosing unexplained weight loss:

- For suspected gastrointestinal problems, such as

malabsorption disorders, inflammatory bowel disease, or celiac disease, consult a gastroenterologist.

- **Endocrinologists:** To assess hormonal imbalances, such as diabetes, thyroid conditions, or dysfunction of the adrenal glands.

- **Oncologists:** When cancer is detected, oncologists will help with additional testing, diagnosis, and treatment planning.

An extensive patient history and physical examination are the first steps in the complex process of diagnosing unexplained weight loss. To determine the underlying reason, imaging scans, blood tests, and expert evaluations are frequently required. A multidisciplinary team comprising experts, psychologists, and nutritionists is frequently necessary to properly identify and address the underlying reason of inexplicable weight loss. Determining the cause early on is essential to avoiding more health issues and giving the patient the right care.

CHAPTER 8

Lifestyle Factors' Effects

Body weight is significantly influenced by lifestyle variables. Particularly, unexplained weight loss is frequently caused by a variety of aspects of a person's everyday life, such as their level of physical activity, sleep patterns, eating habits, and substance usage. With an emphasis on spotting small adjustments that could aid in weight loss, this chapter examines how these lifestyle factors interact with hunger, metabolism, and general health to affect weight. For both patients and healthcare professionals looking to address unexplained weight changes, it is essential to comprehend these issues.

8.1 Weight and Physical Activity Levels

Body weight is significantly impacted by physical activity, which affects metabolism and energy expenditure. It is crucial to comprehend how variations in activity levels might result in inexplicable weight changes, even though the majority of people link physical exercise to weight reduction or maintenance.

A rise in physical activity

Increased physical activity can occasionally lead to inadvertent weight loss, particularly if it occurs suddenly or intensely. This could happen via a number of mechanisms:

- High levels of physical activity result in an increase in the number of calories burnt throughout the day. People may experience a negative energy balance and lose weight if they don't make up for this increase by eating more food.

- **Muscle Mass:** Excessive or strenuous activity, particularly when combined with a poor diet, might cause muscle loss instead of fat loss. Even if there is not a considerable decrease in body fat, this can still lead to total weight loss. This is especially true for athletes who overtrain or participate in endurance training without getting enough sleep or recuperation.

- **Overtraining Syndrome:** When people exercise too

much without allowing their bodies enough time to recuperate, they may develop overtraining syndrome (OTS). Fatigue, hormone abnormalities, decreased appetite, and inexplicable weight loss are some of the consequences. Stress triggers changes in the body's metabolism, which can have a big impact on weight.

Reduction in Exercise

Conversely, weight changes can also result from abruptly reducing physical activity, however these are usually linked to weight gain rather than loss. However, inactivity can aid in weight loss when paired with other elements like bad eating patterns or mental health conditions by:

- **Muscle Atrophy:** Muscle atrophy is frequently the result of inactivity. A decrease in muscle mass over time may result in a drop in the body's basal metabolic rate (BMR), which may impact total body weight by causing a loss of lean tissue.
- A sedentary lifestyle may be a contributing factor to disturbances in hunger signals and appetite regulation, which can result in a decreased appetite.

Less physical activity might cause people to feel less hungry, which could result in unintended weight loss if they aren't eating enough to meet their body's demands.

Points to Keep an Eye on

Unexpected weight loss may indicate a change in the ratio of energy intake to expenditure in any scenario, regardless of whether activity levels are rising or falling. When determining the underlying causes of weight loss, medical professionals will take into account variables including the kind, frequency, and intensity of physical exercise as well as the existence of any symptoms like exhaustion or decreased appetite.

8.2 Eating and Sleep Patterns

Sleep is essential for controlling hunger, metabolism, and total weight. The hormone balance that governs appetite, satiety, and energy expenditure can be upset by irregular eating patterns and poor sleep patterns, which can lead to inexplicable weight loss. The impact of sleep and eating schedule interruptions on weight will be discussed in this subchapter.

Anomalous Sleep Habits

It has been demonstrated that sleep deprivation or poor sleep quality significantly affects weight regulation. The hormonal balance of the body is impacted by disturbed sleep patterns, which can result in changes in metabolism and hunger. Among the main areas impacted by inadequate sleep are:

- **Hormonal Disruption:** Lack of sleep can lead to an imbalance in hormones that control hunger, including leptin, which indicates fullness, and ghrelin, which increases appetite. Long-term sleep loss tends to raise ghrelin and lower leptin, which increases appetite and encourages overeating. However, the body may react to extreme sleep disturbance by reducing hunger, particularly if the person feels overly exhausted.

- **Stress Response:** Sleep deprivation raises the stress hormone cortisol, which affects hunger and metabolism. Over time, catabolism—the breakdown of muscles—caused by elevated cortisol levels may help people lose weight.

- **Metabolism Slowdown:** Lack of sleep impairs insulin sensitivity, which causes problems with the body's glucose metabolism. This can lead to weariness, decreased exercise, and changed calorie consumption, which can help people lose weight, especially those who already have metabolic disorders.

Unusual Eating Patterns

Another important factor in controlling weight is eating habits. The following factors may put people who have inconsistent or irregular eating patterns such as missing meals, eating late, or emotional eating at risk for inexplicable weight loss:

- **Disrupted Metabolism:** The body's circadian cycle, which controls metabolic functions, might get confused by irregular meal timings. The body may find it difficult to appropriately control appetite and energy expenditure when meals are skipped or consumed at irregular times, which could result in either overeating or undereating at the wrong periods.

- **Digestive Issues:** Unusual eating habits might cause discomfort in the digestive tract, which can impact appetite. Inconsistent eating patterns can exacerbate conditions like indigestion, bloating, and acid reflux, which can deter regular eating and lead to weight loss.

- **Nutritional Deficiencies:** Poor dietary choices or meal skipping can lead to inadequate nutritional intake, which can cause deficiencies that cause inadvertent weight loss. Muscle function and general metabolic health can be negatively impacted by a lack of protein, vitamins, and minerals.

Points to Keep an Eye on

Weight may be impacted by inconsistent sleep or eating patterns if you experience symptoms like weariness, irritability, frequent hunger, or a decreased appetite. Finding lifestyle factors that can be causing weight loss requires keeping an eye on the regularity of mealtimes and sleep schedules.

8.3 Drug Abuse and How It Affects Weight Changes

Smoking, drinking, and using drugs are among the substances that can have a major impact on body weight through a number of mechanisms, such as altered digestion and metabolism or appetite suppression. Unintentional weight loss can result from these drugs' direct and indirect effects, and in certain situations, the loss can be severe.

Smoking

Weight loss is frequently linked to cigarette smoking, especially for heavy smokers. The primary component of tobacco, nicotine, is a stimulant that has a variety of effects on the body.

- Nicotine has been shown to decrease appetite, especially by raising norepinephrine levels in the brain, which can suppress hunger. Smokers may consume less, which could result in weight loss and an energy deficit.

- **Increased Metabolism:** Nicotine also increases the pace at which calories are burned by the body. Over time, this increase in energy expenditure may help people lose weight, particularly if they don't modify their calorie intake to make up for it.

- Smoking can impair gastrointestinal function by slowing down digestion, lowering blood flow to the stomach, and raising the risk of peptic ulcers. These effects can result in decreased nutrient absorption and weight loss.

Drinking Alcohol

Chronic alcohol use and weight have a complicated relationship, but because it affects appetite, digestion, and nutritional absorption, it may occasionally help people lose weight:

- Alcohol has the ability to both increase and decrease appetite, which can result in irregular eating habits. Chronic drinkers may choose to eat unhealthy foods or skip meals, which might result in inadequate nutrition.

- **Caloric Imbalance:** Drinking alcohol can lead to weight gain because it contains empty calories, or calories that have no nutritious value. On the other hand, weight loss brought on by liver illness, alcohol-induced nausea and vomiting, or starvation can also result from heavy alcohol usage.

- **Liver Dysfunction:** Cirrhosis, alcoholic liver disease, and liver failure are among the conditions that can result from excessive alcohol consumption. Significant weight loss may result from these disorders since they interfere with metabolism and impede the intake of nutrients.

Substance Abuse

By altering hunger, digestion, and metabolism, several prescription and recreational medicines can also affect weight. Typical medications associated with weight reduction include:

- **Stimulants:** Cocaine and methamphetamine are well-known for reducing hunger and speeding up the metabolism. People who use these medications may lose weight quickly and significantly.

- **Opioids:** Prolonged use of opioids, such as heroin and prescription medicines, can result in weight loss because of nausea, constipation, and appetite reduction, even if they may initially produce weight gain.

- **Antidepressants and Chemotherapy:** Some drugs used to treat cancer or depression can produce nausea, altered appetite, and gastrointestinal problems, all of which can lead to weight loss.

Points to Keep an Eye on

In cases of unexpected weight loss, substance use should be carefully considered. To find out how these factors might be causing weight changes, healthcare professionals will ask about drug, alcohol, and tobacco use as well as any changes in consumption patterns.

Body weight regulation is greatly influenced by lifestyle factors, such as sleep patterns, eating habits, substance use, and physical activity levels. A number of physiological and behavioral factors, including both increased and decreased physical activity, sleep deprivation, irregular eating patterns, and substance use, can lead to inexplicable weight loss. By knowing how these factors affect weight, people can make well-informed decisions about changing lifestyle choices that might be causing undesired weight changes, and medical professionals can provide tailored guidance and interventions to help people control their weight.

CHAPTER 9

MANAGING AND TREATING INEXPLICABLE WEIGHT LOSS

Unexpected weight loss is a complicated medical condition that needs to be managed and treated with a multifaceted, all-encompassing strategy. Understanding the underlying causes of weight loss and collaborating with medical practitioners, nutritionists, and mental health specialists are essential to properly addressing this issue. This chapter explores the methods used to treat and manage inexplicable weight loss, emphasizing dietary changes, medical and psychological interventions, and the value of continuous observation and follow-up.

9.1 Nutritional Assistance and Dietary Modifications

Personalized nutritional support and dietary modifications are essential for dealing with inexplicable weight loss. Nutritional therapy aims to help patients regain a healthy weight and enhance their general well-being, regardless of the cause of their weight loss—be it a medical condition, lifestyle choices, or psychological problems. Dietitians are essential to this process because they collaborate closely with patients to create customized meal plans that meet their unique dietary requirements and preferences.

The Dietitian's Role:

In order to identify and treat any underlying dietary deficits that might be causing weight loss, dietitians are crucial. They evaluate the patient's food, spot any irregularities, and create a customized dietary plan. Usually, the procedure entails:

- **Comprehensive Assessment:** The dietitian thoroughly examines the patient's medical history, eating habits, and weight loss trends. This entails being aware of the kind and quantity of food being ingested, any gastrointestinal problems, allergies, or sensitivities, as well as other lifestyle elements like stress and physical activity.

- **Nutritional Diagnosis:** The dietitian may identify

nutritional imbalances or deficiencies (such as poor vitamin and mineral intake, protein inadequacy, or inadequate caloric intake) that may be causing weight loss based on the evaluation.

- **Education and Meal Planning:** A customized meal plan is created to make sure the patient gets enough calories and nutrients to reach a healthy weight again. To treat deficiencies and provide a balanced intake of vitamins, minerals, and macronutrients (proteins, carbs, and fats), the dietitian may suggest particular meals or supplements.

Dietary Techniques for Regaining Weight

Dietitians concentrate on methods that support patients' weight growth in a sustainable and healthful way. These tactics frequently consist of:

- Dietitians may suggest nutrient-dense foods, which are high in calories but low in volume, such as avocados, nuts, seeds, and full-fat dairy products, to patients who are having trouble eating enough to maintain or regain weight. These meals give the patient the number of calories they need without being too heavy.

- **Frequent, Smaller Meals:** Having smaller, more frequent meals throughout the day can assist enhance caloric intake in people who have trouble eating large meals. Dietitians could recommend a regimen that consists of several easy-to-eat snacks, smoothies, or liquid meals.

- **Fortified Foods:** Dietitians may also suggest including foods high in calories in regular meals. For instance, adding nut butters, oils, or powdered milk to soups, smoothies, or casseroles can raise their calorie content without needing significant dietary adjustments.

- Dietitians will collaborate with gastroenterologists to offer foods that are easier to digest, or they may recommend the use of digestive enzymes or other supplements, in cases when weight loss is caused by digestive problems (such malabsorption).

Personalized Dietary Interventions

Personalization is the key to weight restoration success. Dietitians strive to comprehend the particular requirements, inclinations, and health issues of every patient. For instance, a patient who is losing weight because of cancer might need different nutritional strategies (such as calorie-dense, high-protein meals and soft, easily digestible foods) than someone who is losing weight because of a chronic illness or mental health condition. The objective is to create a plan that is in line with the patient's health objectives and sustainable.

9.2 Treatments in Medicine and Psychology

Addressing the underlying medical and psychological issues is frequently necessary when managing unexplained weight loss. These treatments might include psychiatric therapy intended to address emotional and mental health concerns that may be influencing appetite and food consumption, as well as medical procedures targeted at treating certain illnesses.

Medical Interventions for Comorbidities

Unexpected weight loss is frequently a sign of a disease like cancer, gastrointestinal issues, thyroid issues, or persistent infections. Weight stabilization or restoration may result from the right medical treatments that are started to manage or alleviate the illness process after the underlying issue has been detected. Typical medical strategies include of:

- **Pharmacological Treatments:** Drugs may be recommended to control hormone levels and metabolic processes in diseases such as diabetes or hyperthyroidism. Drugs like corticosteroids or immune-suppressants may be used to treat inflammation and enhance nutrient absorption in situations of gastrointestinal disorders like Crohn's disease.

- **Cancer Treatments:** Chemotherapy, radiation, or targeted therapy are important ways to manage the underlying disease in individuals who have cachexia, or weight loss, which is a side effect of cancer. To assist boost appetite, doctors may also prescribe appetite stimulants like corticosteroids or megestrol acetate.

- **Surgical Interventions**: Surgery may be required to address the underlying cause and enhance nutritional intake when unexplained weight loss is brought on by gastrointestinal blockages, malabsorption, or other problems that call for surgical correction.

Psychological Interventions for Weight Loss Associated with Mental Health

Mental health conditions like despair, anxiety, eating disorders (such anorexia nervosa), or long-term stress are frequently linked to unexplained weight loss. Thus, psychological therapies are a crucial component of the management strategy. Important therapies consist of:

Cognitive behavioral therapy, or CBT, is a very successful treatment for mood and eating problems that lead to weight loss. Its main goal is to alter harmful cognitive patterns and actions associated with eating, body image, and self-worth. CBT promotes better eating habits and assists patients in challenging skewed beliefs about food and weight.

Patients whose weight loss is associated with anxiety, stress, or sadness may benefit from psychotherapy to address underlying emotional problems. Stress management, mindfulness, and relaxation techniques are among methods that can assist lessen the emotional triggers that might be influencing hunger.

In order to address any dysfunctional patterns within the family that might be influencing the patient's eating behaviors and weight loss, family therapy may be required in cases of eating disorders.

Psychological Support Medication

Medication may occasionally be used to treat mental health conditions that are causing weight loss. Patients may find it easier to eat enough food if they use antidepressants, anxiety drugs, or appetite stimulants to assist control their mood and appetite. Antidepressants like bupropion and selective serotonin reuptake inhibitors (SSRIs) can help stabilize mood and increase energy, which may have a good impact on eating behaviors.

9.3 Observation and Monitoring

For patients to successfully manage unexplained weight loss and return to a healthy weight, routine monitoring and follow-up care are essential. This phase of treatment is crucial for evaluating results, spotting side effects, and modifying treatment regimens as necessary.

The Value of Consistent Monitoring

In order to measure weight, evaluate nutritional intake, and make sure treatment regimens are working, patients who are losing weight for no apparent reason need to be monitored continuously. Frequent check-ins assist medical professionals in identifying any alterations in the patient's state and averting consequences. Monitoring ought to consist of:

- **Weight Tracking:** To track the pace of weight growth or decrease, regular weigh-ins are necessary. This aids medical professionals in assessing the efficacy of the current course of treatment and identifying areas for improvement. In certain situations, during the initial phases of treatment, patients might be weighed more frequently (weekly, for example).

- Dietitians or nutritionists may do follow-up nutritional assessments to make sure the patient is getting enough calories and nutrients. Food diaries, blood tests for nutritional deficiencies, and recurring assessments of the patient's eating patterns and lifestyle modifications are a few examples of these examinations.

- Regular laboratory testing is necessary to check vital factors that may be impacted by weight reduction, such as liver, kidney, and electrolyte balance. To make sure dietary requirements are being satisfied, blood testing may also measure protein, vitamin, and mineral levels.

Modifying Therapy Programs

Treatment plan modifications can be required if weight loss continues after initial measures. This might entail:

- **Medication Changes:** To make sure a patient is getting enough nutrients, changes may be required if they are taking drugs that impact appetite or weight. This could entail switching prescription drugs, introducing appetite suppressants, or investigating alternative therapy modalities.

- Dietitians may suggest more aggressive nutritional therapies, such as adding high-calorie supplements or looking into different feeding techniques, such as enteral feeding (tube feeding) or parenteral nutrition (IV nutrition), if weight restoration is not improving.

- **Further Diagnostic Testing:** Additional testing could be necessary to rule out conditions that were not previously identified if the underlying cause of unexplained weight loss is still unknown.

Long-Term Care and Recurrence Prevention

Patients require ongoing treatment even after their weight has been restored in order to maintain a stable weight and to continue managing any underlying medical issues. This could entail:

- **Continuous Monitoring:** To avoid further weight loss, follow-up appointments with medical professionals, frequent nutritional evaluations, and ongoing weight monitoring are required.

- **Lifestyle Support:** Maintaining a healthy weight over time requires promoting long-term, good eating practices, exercise, and stress reduction techniques.

- **Mental Health assistance:** To avoid recurring problems like eating disorders, anxiety, or depression that could cause weight loss in the future, patients whose weight loss is related to psychological reasons need to get continuous mental health assistance.

An all-encompassing strategy is needed to manage and treat unexplained weight loss, including dietary changes, medical and psychological interventions, and continuous observation. Patients can successfully regain their health and reach a healthy weight by collaborating closely with a team of medical doctors, nutritionists, and mental health specialists. Both the present problem and the patient's long-term health can be addressed with individualized treatment, frequent check-ups, and an emphasis on the underlying causes of weight loss.

<h1 style="text-align:center">CHAPTER 10</h1>

<h2 style="text-align:center">PROACTIVE HEALTH STRATEGIES AND PREVENTION</h2>

A proactive, all-encompassing strategy is needed to prevent inexplicable weight loss and to promote general well-being. The significance of identifying early warning indicators, establishing a solid support system, and adopting a holistic approach to health is emphasized in this chapter. People can maintain a healthy weight, lower their chance of accidental weight loss, and improve their long-term mental, emotional, and physical health by using these strategies.

10.1 Identifying Warning Signs in Advance

Early identification is one of the best strategies to avoid the detrimental health effects of inexplicable weight loss. Early detection of unwanted weight loss is essential for spotting underlying health problems before they worsen. This section will go over the typical warning indicators that could point to inadvertent weight loss and when people should get help from a doctor.

Preliminary Signs of Inadvertent Weight Loss

Weight loss that cannot be explained usually happens gradually, but there are a few warning signals. People should be conscious of any changes in their bodies that could be signs of an issue. Typical warning indicators include the following:

- **Unexplained Decrease in Appetite:** Weight loss may be evident if there is a marked decrease in appetite that persists for weeks or months. This could indicate an underlying medical illness, including gastrointestinal disorders or infections, or it could be the result of psychological problems, like anxiety or depression.

- **Weakness and exhaustion:** Especially when accompanied by weight loss, persistent weakness or exhaustion may be a sign of thyroid problems, malnourishment, or more severe illnesses including cancer or chronic sickness.

- **Digestive Disturbances**: Weight loss with bloating, stomach pain, or changes in bowel habits (e.g., diarrhea or constipation) may indicate gastrointestinal disorders including Crohn's disease, celiac disease, or malabsorption syndromes.

- **Muscle Wasting or Loss of Strength:** Even if weight loss is not severe, a loss of muscle mass or a sense of weakness could be a sign of a problem with protein intake, nutrient absorption, or an underlying illness like cancer or muscle wasting disorders.

- **Changes in Skin, Hair, and Nails:** Skin, hair, and nail appearance are frequently impacted by unexplained weight loss. For instance, brittle nails, dry skin, and thinning hair may indicate thyroid disorders, vitamin or mineral deficits, or starvation.

- **Persistent Infections or Illness:** Frequent infections, fevers, or unexplained illnesses that cause weight loss could indicate persistent infections like HIV/AIDS or tuberculosis or problems with the immune system.

When to Get Help from a Doctor

Even though some weight loss may be gradual or the result

of transient circumstances (such stress or a minor illness), it is imperative to speak with a healthcare provider if:

- Weight loss that surpasses 5% of total body weight in a brief amount of time (usually within 6 months).
- An inexplicable decrease of appetite that lasts for weeks is present.
- Unexplained weakness or exhaustion makes it difficult to go about regular tasks.
- Complementary symptoms include fever, stomach ache, or trouble swallowing.

Early consultation with a healthcare professional can help guarantee that any underlying psychological or medical conditions are swiftly addressed, thereby averting more catastrophic difficulties.

10.2 Establishing a Network of Support

Having a solid support system is essential for preserving general health and avoiding inexplicable weight loss. The resources, accountability, and encouragement required to manage health and well-being can be obtained with the help of friends, family, and medical experts. The significance of establishing and maintaining a support system for the prevention and treatment of weight loss-related problems will be discussed in this section.

The Function of Friends and Family

An individual's health can be greatly impacted by having a network of friends and relatives who are supportive. Family members can assist by:

- **Tracking Changes:** Family and friends can be extremely helpful in tracking changes in weight, eating patterns, and general health. They might pick up on signs that the person would miss, such decreased appetite, inexplicable exhaustion, or physical changes like weight fluctuations or muscle loss.

- **Offering Emotional Support:** Mental health conditions like anxiety or depression can occasionally be connected to weight reduction. Friends and family may assist a person emotionally, promote good habits, and lessen stress in their lives.

When needed, they can also assist in facilitating access to mental health specialists.

- **Encouraging Healthy Eating:** Promoting balanced eating practices can be greatly aided by social support. Family members can help with grocery shopping, meal planning, and cooking wholesome meals, ensuring that the person gets the nutrients they need to maintain a healthy weight.

- **Encouraging Physical Activity:** Regular physical activity, like yoga, swimming, or walking, can help preserve muscle mass, stop additional weight loss, and enhance general health.

The Function of Medical Professionals

In order to prevent and manage inexplicable weight loss, medical professionals such as physicians, nutritionists, and mental health specialists are essential. They offer professional advice, diagnosis, and alternatives for treatment, such as:

- **Medical Monitoring and Guidance:** By using physical examinations and diagnostic tests, a medical professional can determine the underlying reasons for inexplicable weight loss. They can keep an eye on any illnesses that might be causing weight loss and try to treat them appropriately.

- **Nutritional and Dietary Support:** Dietitians are very helpful in developing customized meal plans to help patients keep a healthy weight. Depending on the patient's demands, they can provide guidance on nutrient-dense diets, supplements, and methods to increase calorie intake.

- **Mental Health Support:** Psychologists and therapists can help with eating disorders, anxiety, and depression, among other psychological issues that may be causing weight loss. Patients who struggle with negative thought patterns that affect their connection with food and body image can benefit from therapy.

Creating an All-Inclusive Support Network

Working together with trusted loved ones and specialists, a complete support network makes sure that all facets of health are taken care of. In order to create a network of support, people should:

- **Involve a Healthcare Team:** Develop a complete treatment plan that is suited to the needs of the individual by collaborating with a group of medical experts, such as a physician, dietician, therapist, and perhaps a personal trainer.

- **Seek Social Support Groups:** Taking part in online or in-person social support groups can give people a feeling of belonging. Support groups for chronic illnesses, mental health, or weight control provide information, emotional connections, and shared experiences.

10.3 Adopting a Holistic Perspective on Medicine

In order to attain overall health, a holistic approach to health integrates mental, emotional, and physical well-being. Adopting a balanced lifestyle is crucial for long-term health maintenance and the prevention of various chronic problems, in addition to preventing inexplicable weight loss. The ways that a holistic approach promotes optimal health and can work as a successful weight loss prevention strategy will be discussed in this section.

Keeping Physical Health in Balance

Maintaining weight is significantly influenced by physical health, which is essential to overall well being. Among the essential elements of physical health are:

- Exercise on a Regular Basis: Regular exercise maintains muscle mass, improves cardiovascular health, and controls metabolism. Whether it be strength training, flexibility exercises like yoga, or cardiovascular activities, exercise may be customized to meet the needs of each individual.

- Maintaining a healthy weight requires eating a balanced diet full of proteins, healthy fats, vitamins, minerals, and carbohydrates. This is known as adequate nutrition. A healthy diet gives you the energy you need for everyday tasks, promotes body processes, and helps avoid nutrient deficits.

- The beginning of significant illnesses that may contribute to weight loss can be avoided by routine health examinations, screenings, and vaccines. Early detection of health problems is ensured by preventive care, allowing for prompt management prior to weight loss.

Emotional and Mental Health

Weight management and physical health are strongly impacted by mental and emotional well-being. Better decision-making, healthier lifestyle choices, and a general sense of well-being are all influenced by a healthy mental and emotional state. Important elements of mental and emotional well-being include:

- **Stress Management:** Prolonged stress can have a detrimental impact on weight, digestion, and appetite. It is possible to control stress levels and avoid weight-related problems by engaging in stress-reduction practices like journaling, deep breathing, meditation, or mindfulness.

- **Emotional Balance:** Maintaining a healthy weight and eating well are related to emotional well-being. A healthy relationship with food and one's body can be achieved by addressing emotional eating, trauma, and body image issues through therapy or self-care techniques.

- **Social Connections**: Creating and preserving deep connections with people offers a sense of belonging and emotional support, both of which enhance general wellbeing. Additionally, social connections can lessen depressive or lonely sentiments, which might contribute to weight loss.

Long-Term Health Lifestyle Decisions

Making deliberate, constructive lifestyle decisions that promote long-term health is a key component of taking a holistic approach. These options consist of:

- **Adequate Sleep:** Sleep is necessary for hormone balance, weight control, and recuperation. To guarantee that the body can relax, recover, and sustain ideal metabolic function, aim for 7-9 hours of sleep per night.

- **Hydration:** Maintaining a healthy metabolism and digestion requires adequate hydration. Dehydration, which can result in weariness, poor vitamin absorption, and digestive problems, can be avoided by drinking enough water.

- **Avoiding Harmful Substances:** Reducing or quitting the use of drugs, alcohol, or tobacco for recreational purposes can have a major positive impact on one's physical and mental well-being. Weight loss and other health issues may result from these drugs' interference with appetite, metabolism, and food absorption.

Long-Term Strategies for Wellness

A holistic approach to health is a sustained effort rather than a quick remedy. In order to preserve good health and avoid inexplicable weight loss, people should:

- **Make Minor, Long-Term Adjustments:** Prioritize long-term, sustainable lifestyle adjustments over short-term, severe diets or workout regimens. Long-term health maintenance requires consistency.

Cultivate Mindful Living: Pay attention to the decisions you make every day about your diet, level of activity, and emotional health. Being aware can assist people in making deliberate decisions that promote general well-being.

- **Make self-care a priority:** Frequent self-care activities, such hobbies, relaxation, and time for introspection, lower stress and enhance general wellbeing.

A holistic approach to health ensures long-term vitality and quality of life by empowering people to take charge of their health and preventing unexplained weight loss.

ABOUT THE AUTHOR

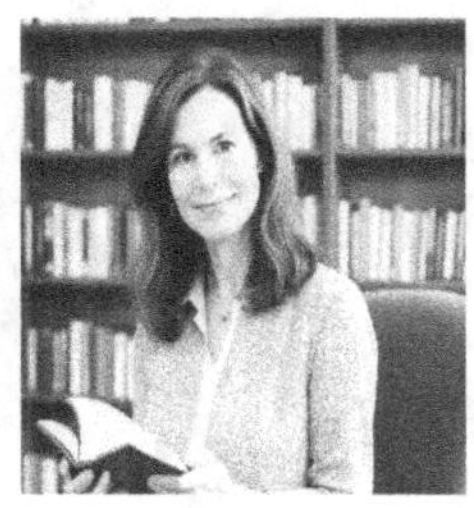 Sophia Royce Smartwell is a committed writer who specializes in wellness and health, offering insightful information on mental and physical health. She is deeply passionate about educating readers on important health issues and trying to close the knowledge gap between medical research and common sense. Her publications are designed to give people the knowledge they need to take charge of their health in an understandable, approachable, and evidence-based manner.

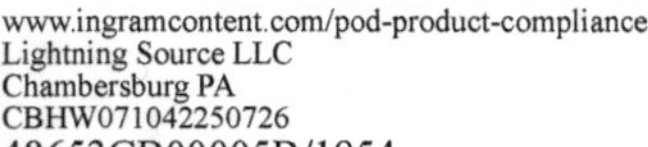